Community Chest

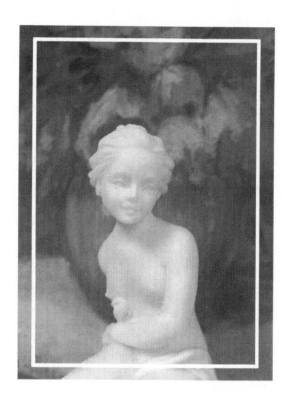

Natalie Serber

Two Sylvias Press

Two Sylvias Press
PO Box 1524
Kingston, WA 98346
twosylviaspress@gmail.com

Cover Design: Kelli Russell Agodon
Book Design: Annette Spaulding-Convy
Author Photos: Deena Hofstad

Created with the belief that *great writing is good for the world*, Two Sylvias Press mixes modern technology, classic style, and literary intellect with an eco-friendly heart. We draw our inspiration from the poetic literary talent of Sylvia Plath and the editorial business sense of Sylvia Beach. We are an independent press dedicated to publishing the exceptional voices of writers.

To learn more about Two Sylvias Press, please visit:
www.twosylviaspress.com

ISBN-13:978-0692492598
ISBN-10:0692492593

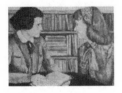

Two Sylvias Press
www.twosylviaspress.com

Praise for *Community Chest*

I loved Natalie Serber's smart, funny and bittersweet report from the Land of Breast Cancer. Fear and grief take turns with an "almost normal day"; kindness and honesty collide with "irrational" rage. While generously detailing the unique aspects of her personal journey, she also manages to honor the collective experience so many (too many!) of us have shared. Now we have this story to share too.

—**Elizabeth Rosner**, author of *Electric City*, *Blue Nude*, and *The Speed of Light*

ဆ

Natalie Serber is the kind of friend you long for when things get hard—tough enough to see how dark things can get, but with enough pluck and fortitude to show you how to thrash through it. This perfect memoir is not just a tale of surviving a diagnosis but of truly experiencing it, observing it, and feeling all that it brings—gravity, absurdity, craziness, fury, tenacity, and love.

—**Robin Romm**, author of *The Mercy Papers* and *The Mother Garden*

ဆ

What I loved about this book: the honesty, the unadorned reality, the bitter, the sweet, the surrender—the lucidness, and lyric grace that touched these pages, calling you friend, whispering secrets, helping readers grapple with their own struggles with the fear and pain and shame that comes from a diagnosis of Cancer. Natalie Serber is a born writer, braiding past, present and future into a story that is both vulnerable and strong, witty and filled with insight.

—**Naseem Rakha**, author of *The Crying Tree*

୬

Natalie Serber's *Community Chest* closely describes and considers her experience of breast cancer—from diagnosis through surgery and chemotherapy and recovery to the lovely abyss of remission. Serber's prose is totally stunning, is both clipped, compact and capaciously expansive. The writing reveals Serber's varied emotional, bodily experience with great precision and complexity. She especially writes deeply about the experiences of loneliness and anxiety (*Anxiety is imagining forward, imagining the worst.*). The knockout sections here are "Pierced" and "#Baldunderneath." Both describe what underscores any day of illness (any day of wellness too)—loss of body, decline of the body amidst other bodies in decline, in fruition, and even though Serber experiences (and endures) bodily loss, the prose forms into its own beautifully fecund body regaining itself.

—**Jay Ponteri**, author of *Wedlocked* and *Darkmouth Strikes Again*

Acknowledgements

Many people showed up to help see me through. I am grateful to the medical professionals, Dr. Jennifer Garreau, Dr. Robert Raish, Dr. Regan Look, Dr. Stephanie Anderson, thank you for expertise and your many kindnesses. To the staff at Compass Oncology, I am grateful for your warmth. To Ella Roggow, thanks for holding my hand and for listening. Denise Gour, thank you for your calm comfort. And to Barbara D. Johnson, Sarah Sentilles, Laurel Graham, Peggy Merchant, Jennifer Thomas, Jay and Amy Ponteri, Maureen Moran, Nancy Hales, friends and neighbors too numerous to list, thanks for keeping my spirits up. To my family, Sarah Hart, Molly Hart and Carole Hart, thanks for your love and support. Mom, I love you. And of course, to Joel, Miles and Sophie, you are everything to me.

Thanks as well to Lee Montgomery, Kelli Russell Agodon and Annette Spaulding-Convy for believing in this manuscript, for your efforts on my behalf and for your smart eyes and open hearts.

Table of Contents

Letter to Reader

I was home alone on a Tuesday morning when my breast surgeon called with the results of my biopsy. I'm sorry, she said. As soon as we hung up, I called a close friend and asked her—in what must have been the tiny, frightened voice of a child—to please come over and sit with me. Of course, she responded, but who is this?

That's what my bad diagnosis did to me. It terrified me. It made me unrecognizable. I was not the person meant to be ill. I was the hand holder, the meal deliverer, the person who sat at a friend's side playing scrabble while the chemo dripped.

My diagnosis also made me feel terribly alone, which is a paradox isn't it? For yes, of course we have to move through the fear, the uncertainty and the suffering alone inside our heads, but suffering and sorrow are part of the human experience. Our particular grief connects us with one another.

My friend rushed over right away in her nightgown; she stumbled up the front porch steps and sat beside me. She was one of many friends and family members who helped to see me through.

If you've received your own bad diagnosis, I hope my story makes you feel less alone. I hope reading about how I made it through makes you feel a little bit stronger. I hope you feel me beside you, seeing you through.

~Natalie Serber

For
Peggy, Gail, Lynne, Lisa Mae, Shelley,
Amy, Cathy, Sarah, Liz, Allison, and Ru—
All sisters and survivors, thank you
for sharing your stories with me.

And, for Roberta Friedman
1957 – 2013

℘

A portion of proceeds from *Community Chest*
will be donated to:

Northwest Hope and Healing, whose mission is to provide financial assistance to women in need who are battling breast and gynecological cancer. The Patient Assistance Fund provides assistance for everyday living expenses, such as child care, groceries, reliable transportation, and emergency rent.

I
The Wrong O

Shortly after my first book was published, I began playing a game with myself. Every time my cellphone lit up and listed "private caller," I paused, took a deep breath, and imagined my literary fairy godmother, Oprah, calling to tell me how much she loved my book—how she laughed and was moved by my sentences and that reading my book made her feel less alone. Usually it was a political campaign calling, requesting more money. Now the game is over. Every time my phone rings and the screen lists "private caller," I take a deep breath because more than likely it will be my oncologist. I've gone from one O to another. . . from the O writers love to hear from to the O nobody wants to hear from. Crap. There really is no other way to say it, except to say it. I've been diagnosed with breast cancer. It sucks. Completely.

The cancer seems like an accident. I was seeing my doctor for minor issue and while I was there, I asked for a breast exam. I believe that if you're ever, ever, ever arm's length away from a pair of trained hands, get a breast exam. Of course, I knew there was nothing wrong, except my doctor lingered too long on the left side. She checked my chart and decided to send me to the breast surgeon. I was okay with that. Ready to get that clean bill of health, right?

At the surgeon's office soothing prints decorated the walls—a bicycle leaning against a fence, a field of lavender, stone bridges crisscrossing a meandering river—all suggestive of a serene European vacation.

Coffee and tea were provided along with baskets of Cremora, red stir sticks, and little pink ribbon pins. A half-round aquarium was tucked in a corner, its cold surface bulging into the room reminded me of a giant breast. The glass was magnified, and the plastic kelp looked mossy and prehistoric. One black fish glided in a terrible orbit, growing small and large, horrifying. I named him Tumor. I could do things like that because I, of course, didn't have breast cancer.

While I waited, I made a few notes in my journal. (I thought all of these details might someday be useful, you know, for a story I would write about someone else.) The music was Christian rock. Lyrics included "What are you going to do when your time has come?" and "Your glory fills the sky." Good thing I don't have cancer, I thought, or this would be really upsetting.

I decided I would only say something about the music to the surgeon if she was not wearing a cross. When she apologized about my lengthy wait, I told her it was fine but for the music. She expressed surprise when I described the playlist, then added, "Usually I'm telling someone they have cancer and Madonna is singing 'Like a Virgin.'" To me, that seemed like a much more hopeful, life-affirming soundtrack.

She examined my breast and recommended an ultrasound and mammogram. Sure, it had only been ten months since my last mammo, but let's err on the safe side, the surgeon said. I was still okay with everything. I still felt positive that it would amount to nothing rather than everything. When I checked into the breast center, instead of the tiny stall I normally get for disrobing from the waist up, they put me in the Four Seasons of dressing rooms, with a phone and a lamp and a box of tissues. Shit.

Now I was scared. Now I wished I had brought my husband. I took a few pictures with my iPhone, thinking I would post them to Facebook and say something about fear and how lucky I felt to be cancer free, and send big love to those who may receive a different diagnosis than the one I was going to get.

The rest of the appointment was an unoriginal terrifying blur. Mammogram. Ultrasound. I remember when I was pregnant and ultrasounds were thrilling. I remember staring at the blurry curled-up bean with the fluttering center, the way the room filled with the swish-swish of the baby's heart. As soon as my technician started clicking, I knew it was bad. That click was the sound of measuring. Once the measuring marked the growth of my babies, now it marked the size of my torment. It marked my future. When I began to cry, the tech brought in the doctor who gently placed her pale hand on my thigh. She told me I would be okay. I told her that depended on her version of okay. I might have gone a little crazy. I told her that if she believed in forty virgins awaiting her in some otherworld glory, then I was not going to be okay.

After the biopsy puncture, I was sent back in for a second mammogram. I was sobbing and the technician said to me, "You'll be okay. A little surgery. A little chemo. A little radiation. You'll be good as new." I wanted to say, Fuck you. Who ever heard of a lil' chemo? Instead, I asked her to please be quiet.

The mammogram tech was the first in a long line of people to say weird things:

I signed up for guitar, French, golf, dressage, knitting, and I have you to thank. (If my diagnosis serves as your carpe diem kick in the ass, well, can you please keep it to yourself?)

So sorry to hear about this. I lost a friend to cancer last year. (I'm sorry for your loss, and you just ratcheted up my fear ten-thousandfold.)

Tell me about your surgery. . . and then, when you do, they cover their mouth in horror. (I know the surgery sounds horrible, but if you don't have the stomach for it, please don't ask. I'm already horrified on my own.)

People mean well, they do, but no one knows exactly what to say. A cancer diagnosis will always be scary. My diagnosis brought people closer to their own mortality. But I refused to be responsible for making someone else feel comfortable with the cancer. I wasn't going to lay my coat down so other people could step over the puddle and keep their shoes dry.

During this early post-diagnosis time, I was on a plane and waiting to use the bathroom. A man came out and I looked into that tiny space. The toilet seat was up. I paused. Sure, sure, I could go in and use a piece of toilet paper to lower his seat, but I thought, no. I have cancer and I'm not responsible for your bad manners. I followed this guy up the aisle and asked him to go back and lower the toilet seat. I might have gone a little crazy. But he did it. He apologized.

People also say lovely things:

I love you.
You will be okay.
We caught it early.
May I hug you?

I am lucky. The cancer was small. I didn't feel lucky. I felt scared. I wanted to send the same big love to myself that I imagined sending to the other women who were, or had, or would be inhabiting that Four Seasons dressing room. Women who must endure the puncture and the wait and the bad phone call. I felt their fear. I felt their sorrow. I wanted to feel their strength because surely they were stronger than me.

I wish I could write about the surgery, but I don't remember much. I don't remember waking up at 5:30, thirsty, but not allowed to drink, slipping on yoga pants and a sweatshirt to drive to the hospital in the rain the same way I remember driving to the hospital in the rain at dusk on a cold February day when I was in labor with our son, how every bump and turn and stop sign ratcheted up my pains, or the way I remember driving to another hospital when I was in labor with our girl, panting hard, squeezing my legs together, clutching the door handle, so excited to hold the baby in my arms. I don't remember parking. I don't remember checking in or if I brought anything with me, like the overnight bag I brought when I delivered our children. I do remember taking a Lorazepam and then feeling so grateful when my nurse gave me another. I remember being wheeled back to the breast center for more imaging, traveling between buildings on the glass sky bridge; the sunrise pink and orange through the windows reminded me of Venice, and I thought I was on my own Bridge of Sighs. The doctor, a gruff white-haired man, was the first person who didn't treat me with kindness. He barely spoke to me, didn't let me know that he was about to stab a long needle into my nipple, twisting and prodding it deep inside, shooting it up with dye or radioactive somethings. . . I quit wanting to know the specific details at some point, it was just too medieval and awful, but I'd have liked a heads-up on this particular pain. I saw the horror in my husband's face as he watched, his eyes squinting, his mouth falling open. I'm not overly sentimental or attached—when I got the diagnosis it felt like I had a tarantula crawling inside my breast, and all I wanted was to *GET IT OFF*, in fact, I wanted them to take the other one, too, to diminish any chance of recurrence—but I felt bad that my breasts, which I'd yearned for at age eleven, which had been groped and caressed, squeezed into lace push-up bras, sunburned, kissed and sucked, which linked me intimately to my infants, which had begun to humorously droop toward my belly, weren't treated a little more gently, with a little more respect. I realized I was thinking of them as a separate entity from me, from the self, but I had to, considering the decision I'd made. And that's all I remember. I know my husband had a stream of visitors while he waited through the lengthy surgery. He promised not to leave the hospital at all. I needed him there, to hold me up with his spirit and love in the same way I sometimes hold up our plane by doing Kegels over the Pacific Ocean. I know that he and our friends cheered and hugged one another when the surgeon came out and told them my lymph nodes were clean. I know that he was by my bed when I awoke.

II
The Situation Room

Four days post-surgery I feel remarkably well-ish. Nights are difficult, but days are slowly improving. My biggest complaint is my muddled brain. A paragraph, no matter how many times I read it, makes little sense. Words elude me. I'm swamped with dismay, anger, sorrow, frustration, apprehension, and amazement—all at once. I know it is arrogant to feel dismay about my diagnosis when statistics say 1 in 8 women will be stricken with breast cancer. What makes me think I could sneak by unscathed? I guess that's how we all get through our days.

I want to make some sense of all this mess, on the page, where I go to make sense of most things in my life. But, my brain is too swimmy. Even my vision is less sharp. I can't believe people take pain medications for fun. I am flotsam on my own couch, awash in pillows and blankets, magazines and remote controls and CNN. I am in the Situation Room with Anderson Cooper and Superstorm Sandy. It is uncanny how much the blurry, radar storm image looks like the ultrasound of my breast and the cancer—the whorl and the eye right there in the lower right portion of the screen. I am stuck, my mind a cable news channel rehashing the same facts—lucky it was found, margins, wind speed, staging, people without power, water level, exploding substations, bilateral mastectomy, sentinel nodes, dusky nipples, proliferation rate, flooded subways, treatment plan. No one knows the level of damage.

The Oregon Symphony called our home in the

hopes I would purchase season tickets. When I told the woman on the phone it wasn't a good time, she asked when would be a good time. I didn't know the answer. In the Situation Room you have to live with negative capability. In art and literature, I love it. In real life, it totally sucks. Not knowing is part of superstorms and cancer. So, you let people take care of you and love you. My surgeon read my book before my surgery. She invited me to her book group. She told me I was singing "Leaving on a Jet Plane" in the operating room, but I don't believe her. My recovery nurse, Jessica, had brown hair and a sweet voice. She asked me to rate my pain from one to ten. My floor nurse, Heather, had clear blue eyes that watched my face for signs of pain. She friended me on Facebook when she got home. I am so lucky. My husband washed my hair. Neighbors put up signs across the street from my house. BIG LOVE and, with a nod toward the title of my story collection, WE SHOUT YOUR LOVELY NAME, NATALIE. Friends brought succulents and flowers and pajamas and magazines and coffee and funny makeup samples, chicken soup, acorn squash soup, split pea soup, bubble bath, lotion, a lovely scarf, tea, candles, novels, elegant dried pears dipped in chocolate, Chinese food, pumpkin pie, and jack-o-lanterns. Web friends reached out, sharing their stories, easing my way.

Today I went for a walk. The leaves are beautiful. My dog barked at his nemesis, Pépé, the Chihuahua from down the street. He's thrilled to bark, to nearly howl. He loves to hate Pépé. It's almost a normal day.

III
Fear of Fear

Without pain medication "on board" my mind is less foggy, and I'm noticing what was and what is no longer. I used to be free to worry (what a strange phrase, *free to worry*, but it's true) about dumb things—our crumbling garden wall, book reviews, squirrels eating all the persimmons, my gray hair, and my thighs. As soon as the ultrasound technician began measuring my lesion with the menacing clicks of her machine, worries gave way to a crushing boulder of fear.

I've never been fearless. When I was a little girl my mom had me wait in the car while she ran in to 7-11 for a quart of milk and a pack of cigarettes. I remember being so anxious about strangers in the parking lot that I hid on the floor behind the driver's seat, closed my eyes and plugged my ears and sang "Kookaburra Sits in the Old Gum Tree." My new fear is immovable, dark and heavy. Singing and hiding won't make it disappear. As I move through my day, I feel it over my shoulder, rolling along, crushing. Sometimes the fear becomes swift, ceaseless hooves in muddy puddles, the thrash and threat of leathery wings. . . I miss my dumb worries. I haven't felt brave for a while.

Fears in no particular order: Death, Loss of Joy, Suffering, Harm to Someone I Love, Cancer, Chemotherapy, Darkness, Silence, Fear. Yes, I'm fearful of being fearful.

I'm trying to shift my perspective. They got it all out. They sliced my tissue razor thin, snooped around, my margins are clean, my nodes are clean. I was walking with a friend the other day. She, too, has had a recent breast cancer diagnosis. She is further along than I am, clean and practically a year out. When I told her about all my pathology, that I am cancer-free, she answered without a moment's pause, "Doesn't feel that way, does it?" Of course she is right, but I am hoping for a day when it does feel that way for both of us. Meanwhile, I am sometimes overcome. Fear is consuming. Fear is molecular. And worst of all, fear is lonely. It starts at the back of my throat. Grips my lungs. I shake. My eyes sting. I feel diminished. I feel stuck. I want to quiet my mind, to cover my eyes, but I am constantly peeping out between my fingers at all the horrible possibilities.

A month after surgery, under the heading of *trying to claim back my life*, my husband and I were intimate for the first time. It was awkward and groping and difficult. The expanders inserted beneath my pectoral muscles felt like giant heads, like Mount Rushmore crushing my chest. My arms could not bear weight. *Ouches, Oh No's, Oh shit, maybe this was a bad idea.*

The day of my biopsy, five weeks earlier, as I stripped down in that Four Seasons dressing room at the breast center, while I was still free to worry, I looked in the mirror at my face and toyed with the idea of Botox. I know, I know, but I thought why not, for the worry creases between my brows, the eleven. Then came the Sturm und Drang of the procedure, the weeping, the pain. When it was over, and I was dressing, the nurse came in and I told her what I'd been thinking about when I arrived, my wrinkles and how decadent that seemed to me now. She said: *Soon enough you'll be free to worry about them again. Free to consider Botox.* I can't wait.

IV
Ding Dong Ditch

No doubt about it, I have been taken down a dark and doorless hallway. I've struggled with fear, discomfort, and abounding messages stating that I am responsible for my own recovery. I get the concept that my attitude will define much of how I endure this ordeal, but I resent it, too. During the treatment decision process, when I wished I had Nate Silver predicting my outcomes and guiding me, I consulted with a radiation doctor who told me, basically, to knock off the sorrow or my prognosis wouldn't be as good. This advice (to put on my big girl panties), delivered only ten days after finding myself in the fearsome teeth of the diagnosis, made me want to. . . well, to punch her in the face. In the end, I was glad for her gruff demeanor, as I did put on my big girl panties and decided I never wanted to be her patient. Her attitude pushed me toward my treatment decisions.

There have also been great generous moments. The universe keeps ringing my doorbell with harbingers of hope. Four nurses shared with me their breast cancer stories. One made a house call, someone I've never before met, to tell me about her surgery. Another offered to show me her reconstructed chest. The generosity bowled me over. She told me to touch her skin and described the lack of sensation that goes hand in hand with her reduced fear of recurrence. On surgery day, one nurse, a powerful She-Ra with long red hair and green eyes, told me that she is ten years out from her diagnosis and then she talked about her grandkids. My acupuncturist told me she doesn't believe in suffering and suggested I drink hot cocoa and continue with the Lorazepam. My GP gave me a troll doll with pink hair and scrubs to keep me company while I recovered. Four weeks after my surgery, I was in New York City for meetings, and a monk walked up to me on Fifth Avenue and gave me a golden *Work smoothly. Lifetime peace* card. (I know it's a scam, but I'm a sap for that kind of thing.) I took my daughter for a facial, and my no-nonsense esthetician took one look at my feet and declared me Russian with strong blood and work to do. She spit through her fingers and knocked on wood.

I am not ashamed to admit that I was susceptible to all of it—the generosity, the serendipity, the kindness, the new age-y, the weird, and the silly. Suddenly, there were so many doors in my dark hallway.

And then, the final surgical pathology came in. The cancer that I'd had, though gone, was particularly strident. The results felt like a gnashing betrayal of all that I'd been reading into the world around me. I would need chemotherapy.

I was a wreck when I went to the patient education session before my first infusion. Walking down the hallway to the conference room door, I brushed my reluctant hand along the wall. My oncologist's nurse, Brittany, caught my eye. When I told her my husband couldn't be there, she stayed with me through the entire session. Patients sitting around a table, each of us with our own particular diagnosis and treatment and white binder outlining side effects and danger signs and things to avoid. Brittany wrote notes in my binder, as if we were seventh grade besties. "I'll get you the right toothpaste.

You'll be fine."

At the end of the session, I found myself alone in the room with a woman I will call Florence. She was perhaps in her late seventies, in a pale-blue velour housedress, still weak and bloated from surgery; she leaned against a pillow that she brought along for comfort. They removed 99% of her tumor, she told me, her chemo was for the remaining 1%. Her eyes were dim, wet, yellow, probably a reflection of my own. I asked her if I could hug her. In that empty room, both of us so afraid, holding each other, I felt another door. How often are we that honest with each other? How often do we let ourselves really just be in the truth? With a stranger? I won't lie, I'm looking forward to joyful truths when this part of my life is behind me, but I also won't deny the power of Florence, of us being humans together.

I would need four chemotherapy infusions, one every three weeks. I would need to see my dentist to make sure my teeth were okay. I might lose my fingernails. I might have trouble with my vein, I might not. I might be nauseous. I might be constipated or suffer from diarrhea. My gums would bleed, my nose would bleed. I might kill my ovaries. I might swell up. I might lose weight. I might become forgetful. I should take baths. I should eat small meals. I should use mouthwash. I should get up and walk around. I should allow myself to rest.

Right away I made a countdown calendar, crossing off the days to the end. Twenty-three days after my first infusion, just as my oncologist predicted, my hair came out in handfuls. It was Christmas Eve. I cried while my husband shaved my head and then our family went out to dinner. Both of my children were also shorn. My son shaved his head the day of my first infusion. He texted me a picture right as the drip started. My daughter cut her hair and sent the long ponytail to Locks of Love to be made into a wig for cancer patients. My husband is bald, so we were a tress-free family. We ate at a fancy-pants restaurant, and we all drank multiple cocktails to blur the elephant at our table. After, all of us tipsy, we went down to the Willamette River, looked across the dark water at the lights of our city, and tossed my hair in.

The infusions took three hours. Whenever the nurses brought over a bag of drugs to hang on a patient's IV pole, they had to dress in hazmat outfits—gloves, extra gowns, masks, and goggles. One of the nurses was pregnant, and I worried about her baby. I was afraid of the slash-and-burn chemo drugs. I was afraid of getting chemo brain. My oncologist told me that yes, chemo brain is real, but so is undernourished, exhausted, stressed, under-oxygenated brain.

And so, every day during my treatment, I walked miles. With family, with friends, with my dog, in the rain, in the cold, and even one day in the snow. It was my own forced march. The whole experience was a forced march punctuated with nosebleeds, digestive problems, sleeplessness, a countertop covered with vitamins and homeopathic remedies, plus nightmares and boring, boring boredom. . . counting the days, watching the drip.

V
Pierced

A couple of months before I received a breast cancer diagnosis, before I was forced to accept in the deepest possible way that I am not in charge, my daughter came home on break from college and showed me in her particular way that I am not in charge.

The morning was chilly, and I stood by her bed in the weak winter sunlight, coffee mug in hand. She opened her eyes and smiled. She's always been a cheerful riser (aside from a brief period of my unhappiness when her hair was pink, and she was pocket-calling me from the beer line at keg parties). As she propped herself up on her elbow, her nightgown, a spring-green acetate shift she'd bought at the Brooklyn Flea Market, the kind of sleepwear pediatricians advise new parents to never, ever let a baby sleep in due to fire safety, slid from her shoulder revealing. . . a pierced nipple.

I might have had an irrational reaction. I withheld the coffee. "You pierced your nipple?"

She yanked the nightgown up.

"You *pierced* your nipple!?!" Thus began my apoplectic rant. In a voice spiraling ever upward, I wondered did she realize she was a poster child for violence against women? Did she know she might never be able to nurse her babies? Did she know what kind of message she might be sending to her intimate partner? That she liked it rough? Oh. My. God. My voice hit its apex. Did she like it rough? I ran down the stairs, yelling out to my husband, "She's pierced her nipple!?!"

He trudged in. Uncertainty, shock, and discouragement scrolled across his face. He was neither upset nor happy with our daughter's choice. He was responding to my reaction. "What am I supposed to do with that information?" he asked.

I ran back upstairs. My daughter calmly told me that she'd used her own money, and it was her body. I cried out, "Flagrant Fucking Foul!" As long as we were paying her tuition, as far as we were concerned (and I may have been using the royal *we* at this point, as my husband was already over it), no money was truly "hers." Moreover, until she was old enough to rent a car, 25, the age of full prefrontal cortex development, her body was only on loan to her. I may have gone a little crazy. I told her that her breast, with the silver spear through it, looked like a canapé at a cannibal cocktail party. I might have yelled this.

"You're insane," she said with excruciating calm as she closed her bedroom door and went back to bed.

Was I? Why had this piercing upset me so much? She hadn't pierced her face again (her nose is pierced and I think it looks great). Her ears are pierced. My ears are pierced, multiple times—well twice in each ear. But her nipple. . . ? Wikipedia says many things about nipple piercing, but the two I glommed onto: "deaths have occurred" and "sexual arousal is enhanced." There you have it. . . sex and death. I wasn't irrational enough to believe she might die from this, but my extreme reaction probably had a bit to do with the fact that her piercing put me face to face with her sexuality, which can be hard for parents, though not for me, I used to think. I have friends who plug their ears and chant *humana, humana,*

humana whenever teens and sex are linked in a sentence. Not a healthy reaction, but an honest one. Face it—sexual activity has psychic and physical ramifications. We cannot follow our children down that baggage-strewn, pothole-ridden-highway. Sure, sure, we can talk about condoms and STDs and emotional impact, but at some point we have to let go.

I saw my daughter's piercing as an act of violence against her breast. Against all breasts. Breasts, for me, represent femininity, a soft sexuality, womanhood, motherhood. I remember how this cherished child of mine once nursed. How she would completely relax, her blue eyes staring up at me until they rolled back as she drifted off into ecstatic slumber.

Of course, breasts can also represent power. When a man claims to be "a breast man," he relinquishes a bit of power to the bearer of those breasts that make him go weak in the knees. But one needn't pierce the breasts to claim the power.

Obviously my feelings are complicated, but at the bottom of it all, I felt assaulted by the violence inherent in the act of piercing. How could she not see that? Maybe what I was really upset about was the possibility that I didn't know my girl. Not in the angry lashing out *I don't even know you* way, but in the potentially heartbreaking *how could we have grown so far apart* way.

The next day, we took a walk. I asked her why she'd done it. She rolled her eyes. I thought that if she had a strong reason—an homage to Robert Mapplethorpe, a take back the breast political statement, an interest in aboriginal body art, I might be able to accept the barbell bisecting her nipple—not like it, but at least be able to grudgingly nod my head.

Here's what she said, "I've wanted to for a long time. It is more interesting than a bellybutton piercing. I don't know."

Here's what I said, "You are nineteen. Your breasts are at their peak. The last thing they need is enhancement."

Here's what she said, "I'm walking home if you keep talking."

Here's what I said, "If it's just a whim, a lark, why not take it out?"

Here's what she said, "No."

What had I done to my body on a lark as a young woman? I'd spritzed on far too much Super Sun-In, turning my brown hair a shocking orange. I endured a frizzled perm. I quit shaving my legs. I once plucked my eyebrows nearly to extinction, leaving a terrible arched tightrope over each eye. My mother's garbled outburst was half-laugh and half-gasp, "What the hell were you thinking?" A good friend of hers, who happened to be in the room with us, said, "They look terrific, honey." They didn't look terrific, but I appreciated the compliment. Could I tell my daughter her nipple looked terrific? For a nanosecond I searched within and came to, No. To me, it looked barbaric. But, guess what, she didn't pierce for my approval. All she wants is for me to get off her back (or her breast) about her choice. What I could do is ask her if it hurt. I could recognize that her choice to pierce isn't a character flaw. I could calm down and accept that she'll be making many choices that don't involve me. I could just be quiet and give her a hug. I love her.

And then came my diagnosis with breast cancer, and the piercing issue became, well, huge. On top of everything else I believed about breasts, turns out they have the potential to kill you. I was suddenly not looking at piercing; I was facing a bilateral mastectomy and then enduring the reconstruction, which would involve expanders, giant syringes, and a second surgery. An experience I would wish on absolutely no one.

The next time my daughter came home from college and I saw the outline of her piercing through her T-shirt, I took it as a full- body slam, as if she had betrayed me and pierced my very heart. Why would she choose to mutilate (my word, not hers) her breast? I begged her to take it out, in solidarity with my struggle. Her piercing became a line of demarcation between us. I'm not saying I was rational, or that cancer-free breasts are too sacred for piercings, but I just felt. . . insulted. The piercing felt flip, cavalier, a dangerous act. My response was part mother hen, as in don't do anything potentially hazardous, like store your cell phone in your bra, and part incredulous and lonely, as in, look how much you can lose; treat your body with the respect it deserves.

My relationship with my own breasts was now far more complicated than before my surgery. After having babies and nursing, I preferred that they not be touched, so losing them was not losing a giant part of my sexuality. I was lucky to have nipple-sparing surgery and a great surgeon. Aside from scars, they look pretty good. The weird results are my feelings of detachment toward my body parts, numbness across my chest and down one arm, as well as the fact that my nipples don't respond to heat or cold. Basically they're like two pink pencil erasers attached to my body. When I complained to my plastic surgeon that I felt like a Victoria's Secret mannequin with my semi-erect nipples, he said, "Isn't that the last thing you'd expect to say after a bilateral mastectomy."

Ouch. . . and, though callous, he's right. But I do miss sensations, the jostling when I run, the tightening across my chest when I swim in the ocean, the softening in the tub.

My daughter claimed that her piercing was a metaphor, which piqued my interest. I love metaphors, but she refused to tell me what it meant. I pondered what a bilateral mastectomy could be a metaphor for. . . giving up the very part of my body that once nourished my children in order to beat back a disease and live my life. In order to claim my life, my body as my own terrain, I had to sacrifice part of it, change its borders. My breasts are gone, and I miss them. When I sleep on my stomach at night, the implants feel hard, inflexibile beneath me. I don't want to hide my heart beneath a shield.

Ultimately, because I ceaselessly pressured her, she took the piercing out. And I felt better, though I think she felt as if she were visiting a police state. If her piercing was a way to claim her body as her own territory, then I was a Viking laying my opinions and values on her.

Writing this all down, I do feel silly about my extreme reaction, and I'm still asking myself why the piercing bothers me so. A friend suggested I might be a bit provincial and should interrogate my prejudices. She said that feigning acceptance of the piercing was a milquetoast response. Yet with our adult children, we have to at least halfway accept things, because as I said at the start of this exploration, we love them, and we are not in charge. Not of our lives or our children's lives. My daughter left home without her piercing whether or not she put it back, I don't want to know. It doesn't really matter. I want to be open and honor my girl's choices.

In the months after my surgery, I thought I should do something bold to reclaim my body from the cancer scare, similar to planting a flag on the moon. Of course now that I have no sensation in my breasts, a pierced nipple seems the perfect gesture, right? Much as I like the irony, I can't do it. Maybe I'll settle for a tattoo.

VI
#BaldUnderneath

A few weeks after my final chemo round, when I began flirting with the idea of giving up my beanies and revealing my aggressively chic inch-long hair growth, I saw a cheerful bald woman eating fish tacos. She took one look at me and said, "I think we have the same hairdresser." I felt downtrodden and walked quickly away.

Anxiety is imagining forward, imagining the worst. When I feel anxious, I ask myself, "Where did you get that information, Natalie?" If the answer is from me, than I say, "Toss it, Smarty. It's not helping you." I'm afraid I don't use a nice tone of voice.

Even in the dark with the chain lock secured across our front door, the steady light from the streetlight shining through our window, our dog snoring at the foot of our bed. Even beneath the quilts, beside the one I love, I can feel terror.

Some people won't show up. I tried not to take it personally. It's about their fear.

Many people surprised me with sweet messages, with finger puppets, hand cream, potted plants, soup, knitted beanies, bubble bath, books and movies.

Eyelashes and eyebrows are useful—they keep debris from falling into your eyes. Without them I looked like a lizard with something in its eye.

Life is not yet the same.

Part of me wanted to be like the bald woman eating fish tacos. . . upbeat, smiling, despite being swollen from the steroids they give with the chemo drugs. Part of me wanted to be nothing like her. I wanted to "pass." I wanted to go out for tacos and not be seen as a cancer patient.

The steroids administered with the chemo drugs really mess you up.

Shitty, shitty, shitty, shitty, shitty, shitty, shitty, shitty, shitty, shitty.

Chemo ≠ waxing. The survivorship counselor told me that a lot of women pay a bundle to be hairless. I paid far too much for this Brazilian.

Isn't there a better word than survivorship?

It's hard to feel lucky, though I know I am.

I have taken aggressive steps to eradicate the disease from my body.

Acupuncture is terrific.

Meditation is hard so I keep trying.

When I first lost my hair, it was an act of bravery to go to the grocery store. Women glanced at me furtively down the cereal aisle. They were trying to discern what about me is different from them. What will keep them safe? I have been one of those women, thinking, I don't smoke, I exercise, I don't eat much meat. None of that kept me safe.

Waking up and going to sleep are times of re-remembering.

Normal is different.

Part of me wanted to smile and hug the bald woman eating fish tacos—to high-five her and say, "We beat it!" Part of me wanted her to go away. I was ashamed of that part of me. I wanted to support her, to connect, but my fear and embarrassment got in the way.

When I was a child I was shocked that there was a zodiac sign called Cancer, and I was so glad I was a Capricorn.

The film *Terms of Endearment* freaked me out.

When my children were little I used to have moments of deep fear of breast cancer, and I would say in my head, *Please, don't let me get cancer. . . at least until the children are in college*. And then the children went to college and I got cancer and I felt prescient, powerful, and that added a new layer of fear.

When I quit dyeing my hair (partly because I was tired of spending the money and partly because I was afraid the chemicals might cause cancer!) and I could barely endure the thatch of slowly growing gray, I thought to myself, I should wait until someday when I have chemo and then let my hair come in gray. Then I'd say, *Stop being so morbid*. Then when I actually needed chemo I was afraid I brought this mess all on myself.

I believe the more I say the word *cancer* the less I will fear it. Psychological pain comes not only from experiences, but also from the words in our heads we use to describe the experiences. Repeating a word like *watermelon* over and over allows the mind to stop associating the sound with the sweet pink flesh and experience it as a meaningless noise.

Cancer, cancer. . .

I have had to face my deepest meaningless noise. I cannot get away from the meaningless noise. NPR sponsors, signs on buses, full-page ads, friends, family members, obits.

I still cannot believe this happened to me. I'm supposed to be the hand-holder.

I am not fierce.

I have less than a 5% chance of recurrence.

I hated it when the radiologist told me I had *baby cancer*.

Baby and cancer should never be said in the same sentence.

I tried to upset the paradigm and view chemo as a pregnancy. A time to be careful, a time that was accomplishing amazing things, a time I would come through and celebrate at the end.

On a bike ride one day, I noticed the breeze against my bare calves. The air felt silky, like swimming past kelp. Days later I realized it was the air rustling baby hairs on my legs, hairs as delicate as lanugo.

Sometimes I want to talk about the cancer and my fear and people get sick of hearing about it. Birth stories are more fun and even they get boring.

Days go so slowly and then suddenly months have passed.

At every new appointment I was given a white binder with useful information. The surgical

oncologist, the oncologist, the infusion center. . .
Even when all the hard treatment work was over
and I began moving toward the next hard part,
survivorship (there's that word again), at my
mindfulness meditation class I was given another
white binder! White binders give me a
stomachache.

Someone asked me if I now "cherish every
moment." I don't know. That seems like a lot of
responsibility. Some moments are kind of shitty.
Some are meh. . . And some, a hug from my
husband, the first sip of coffee in the morning, a
chatty call from my children, a note from a reader,
I do cherish. I do know that I don't want to get
caught in a net of my own worries and concerns. I
know I want to love my family. I know I want to
write. I know I want ease and comfort and
challenge and adventure. Then, the same person
who asked me about cherishing every moment
told me that her friend was having her anus
radiated. I know I feel compassion and concern
for that patient. I know I cherish every moment my
anus is not being radiated.

I wish I could see the bald-fish-taco-eating-lady
today. If I did, I would sit down right next to her
and put the super-spicy salsa on my taco and take
a big bite. I would thank her for reaching out to
me, for making communion with me. We are all
bald underneath.

VII
Getting Current with Myself

At a recent breakfast with two friends, the conversation came around to medical procedures (I know, how middle-aged is that?) as at the table we were a facelift, open-heart surgery, and me. As I listened to my two friends discuss their scars and the remedies they'd used to diminish them, an amazing thing happened—for a moment, and it was a longish moment, I completely forgot that I'd had a bilateral mastectomy. In my head, I was ticking off scars to introduce into the discussion, C-section, a couple of mole removals, and that was it, until, *Oh crap*! I remembered. I suppose I could chalk the omission up to chemo-brain or to the plummeting estrogen that is a by-product of chemo-fried ovaries, but I think it was a moment of me getting current with myself. Yes, I had BC, but the most important word in that sentence was *had*. BC isn't my life.

It's been eight months since my surgery, and four months since my final infusion. Breezy blue skies of summer are starting to make regular appearances here in Oregon, and bright white dogwood blossoms have accepted the spring baton from the now-faded rhododendrons. My hair is beginning to curl away from my scalp, my nose has stopped bleeding, and I feel energized. BC is no longer all-consuming. It isn't my career after all. Turns out it was a really crappy seasonal job, like operating the Tilt-A-Whirl, or standing on the corner of a busy intersection dressed as a giant hamburger waving a foam French fry, or harvesting cantaloupe under a scorching sun.

That isn't to say that I can totally quit, but I won't have all the doctor visits, I won't wake up every morning with my first thought being Cancer (capital letter included). Nor will it be the last thing I consider when I shut my eyes. Before all this happened to me, I would have hesitated even typing the word. Somehow, currently, the power has leached out of it. Sure, sure, I'll be careful about what I consume, what I clean my house with, and the type of shampoo I use (paraben free—yours should be too!), but I will again enjoy a glass of red wine while dicing onions for a marinara sauce. I will tick up my exercise regime, eat tons of mushrooms, kale, and turmeric for their immune-boosting and anti-inflammatory qualities, but I will no longer be quaking.

Not that I will now go through life playing Pollyanna, but I will sweep out my corners. I don't want to carry around niggling disappointments anymore. One thing cancer has taught me is to embark on a path of forgiveness. I thought that would mean starting with the rude flight attendant, then moving on to the acquaintance who needs to be reintroduced to me every time I see her, to the friends (three) who dumped me during my treatment, then, ratcheting up the degree of difficulty like one masters new dives off a springboard, to the disappointing choices my family members sometimes make, and ultimately ending with me. Because really, aren't we all hardest on ourselves?

My therapist wagged her finger at me stating that all that other forgiveness is false if you haven't started with yourself. She asked me to think of myself as a child and offer up some forgiveness to that little brown-haired girl.

Man-oh-man, I hate that kind of thing. It feels silly and fake. But I tried, and the first thing that came to mind was our tiny apartment in Hollywood, California and a dinner party my mom once had. My mom relishes the *party* part of dinner party—the preparing dinner part, not so much. And so, on this particular night, the meal was very late. Her guests, slouched on the wicker couch and in beanbag chairs, seemed unconcerned. Our living room was lit with candles. A heavy cloud of incense, cigarette and pot smoke settled below the equator of the room, and the smell mingled with the spaghetti and meatballs my mother was preparing. Someone ran their fingers through the strings of beads and tiny bells that hung in a doorway. A couple held hands and swayed to the Doors' "Break on Through" and "Hello I Love You." I remember sitting at the coffee table, drawing rabbits in my sketchbook. I was obsessed with rabbits since visiting my Great Aunt Jean and Uncle Bob's farm, where they'd given me two baby bunnies to care for during my stay. My mom's boyfriend stopped strumming his guitar to look over my shoulder and comment on my mastery of the bunny vibe. He pointed to the big rabbit teeth. When dinner was finally ready, my mom called me into the kitchen to help. She'd loaded the platter, sprinkled on Parmesan from the green can. Everyone was at the table, and I was to make the grand entrance bearing the meal. My mother held aside yet another string of doorway beads, and I stepped into the room, tilting the plate just enough to let the entire glorious heap of sauced noodles slide to the floor. There was, of course, a gasp, and then laughter, and then hugs, and rounds of, "Oh, honey" and "It's okay, we'll order pizza." But I was bereft, ashamed. My disappointment in my six-year-old-self was extreme.

Just the fact that I remember the evening so thoroughly, how I ate cornflakes and put myself to bed so miserable at having royally blown my moment of glory, shows how hard I take my missteps. A ton of things can be analyzed out of that evening, but currently the only thing I want to take away is not the atmosphere, the spilling of the pasta, or the grown ups' kindness, but my inability to go easy, to laugh.

Letting go of the bad and opening to the good is made easier by the gradual normalization of my experience. We've all heard the saying *misery loves company* and perhaps rebuked the sentiment because of its schadenfreude aspect. Perhaps *misery needs company* would be more apt. For even though we don't wish suffering on anyone, we don't want to be alone in our pain. Isolation, which is part of the hardship of a cancer diagnosis and treatment, can be debilitating, launching our brains into survival mode, which in turn causes the body to release stress hormones, which can affect our health and contribute to. . . yep, cancer. So indeed, misery needs company. We feel safer in community; relationship reliance is hardwired into our brains from our hunter-gatherer days when being alone in the world meant being prey. Alone = suffering. Community = healing. Thus, I've been building mine. I am a collector of survivor stories. I love hearing of women who are five, ten, twenty years out. I have a doctor friend who works with geriatric patients, and I love to hear the stories of women who forget to mention that BC was part of their past. My friend will be jotting down their medical history, achy hips, high blood pressure, shingles, and then, only upon examination does she discover the BC scars. Other friends and friends of friends have sent me notes letting me know how far out they are from their experience. Angelina Jolie, with her proactive bilateral mastectomy, was another story to collect. Though she did not have breast cancer, she did discover that she carries a gene mutation (BRCA) that makes her susceptible to breast and ovarian cancer; reading the account of her treatment choices in her op-ed in the *New York Times* and the very long chain of comments, was incredibly affirming. Honestly, I haven't been a fan of her films, so I was not swayed by fawning admiration, but I absolutely applaud her decisions, both to undergo the surgery to protect herself and her family and to go public with her story. She has helped countless women, regardless of their BRCA gene status. Her story in her words normalized a treatment option that can make women feel marginalized, freakish, de-sexed. Her piece and the comments it engendered created a community.

A couple of weeks ago, I was flying to New York City again. At the airport I watched women running toward gates and noticed their breasts jiggling. Mine will never do that again. A friend of mine, who had a bilateral mastectomy, told me that after she lost hers, she became obsessed with her daughter's breasts. That song "How Can I Miss You When You Won't Go Away" is true. I rarely thought of breasts, until mine were gone. I also noticed women with hair halfway down their backs and calculated how many years out (what a strange saying, years out. . .) until I would have hair that long. Six? And, here is the best part: the women I noticed who were laughing, chatting on their cell phones, holding hands with a child or a partner, they didn't have anything I didn't have. Yes, the BC took away eight months and body parts, but my joy and confidence are resurging.

Currently, I have two quotes taped to my

bathroom mirror. The first is a Leonard Cohen quote, "The less there was of me, the happier I got." He is referring to his songwriting, but I'm taking out of it whatever I want. The second is from Sonia Sotomayor, "A surplus of effort can overcome a deficit of confidence."

On my flight, I waited in line for the bathroom again. When a man came out and trudged up the aisle toward his assigned seat, I glanced into the tiny room and saw that he'd left the toilet seat up. For a nanosecond I thought about following him and asking him to come back and put it down. Then I decided against it. When it happened the last time I was flying, right after my diagnosis, the stranger's rudeness was just one more thing I couldn't bear. Now, I can.

Postscript

*from my Facebook page
on the anniversary of my diagnosis*

September 27, 2013: One year ago I was having a mammogram that led to an ultrasound that led to the biopsy that led to the diagnosis, surgery, chemo, that led to right now, heading out my door to a yoga class. So grateful to be healthy and energized. I won't lie, part of me is still stunned, frightened. . . but that edge is ebbing away. Women reading this, if you've been putting it off, get a 3D mammogram, and if you have any family history, ask for an ultrasound. Men reading this, encourage your partners, sisters, mothers, and daughters to get screened. #lovethisday

Resources in Portland, Oregon and the Pacific Northwest

Hands On Health
Ella Roggow
www.handsonhealthclinic.com

Compass Oncology
http://compassoncology.com/for-patients/patient-resources/local-resources-support-groups/

Knight Cancer Institute Support Groups
http://www.ohsu.edu/xd/health/services/cancer/getting-treatment/services/support-groups.cfm

Legacy Health Support Groups
http://www.legacyhealth.org/health-services-and-information/health-services/for-adults-a-z/cancer/all-cancer-services/support-groups.aspx

A Mindful Place, Mindfulness Based Stress Reduction
Denise Gour
http://www.mindfulplace.com/index.html

Northwest Hope and Healing/Financial Assistance for Breast and Gynecological Cancer Patients Receiving Treatment at Swedish Medical Center
http://nwhopeandhealing.org

American Cancer Society – Road to Recovery/ Transportation to Treatment
http://www.cancer.org/treatment/supportprogramsservices/app/resource-detail.aspx?resourceId=122326

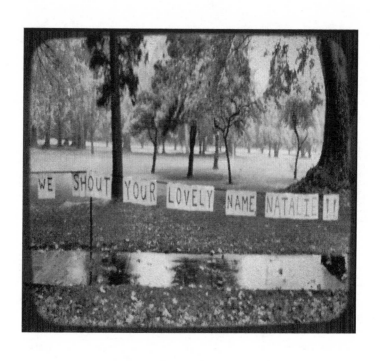

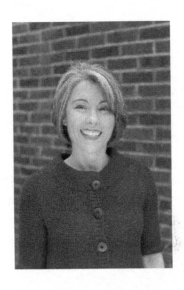

Natalie Serber is the author of the story collection *Shout Her Lovely Name* (Houghton Mifflin Harcourt) a *New York Times* Notable Book of 2012 and a summer reading pick from *O, the Oprah Magazine* and an *Oregonian Top 10 Books of the Pacific Northwest* and an *Indie Next Pick*. Her fiction has appeared in *The Bellingham Review, Gulf Coast, Inkwell,* and *Hunger Mountain*. Her essays and reviews have appeared in, *The New York Times, Salon, The Rumpus, The Oregonian, The San Francisco Chronicle, Fourth Genre,* and *Hunger Mountain*. Awards and grants include the Barbara Deming Grant for Women Artists, Tobias Wolff Award, H.E. Francis Award, John Steinbeck Award, all for fiction, and finalist mentions for the Annie Dillard Creative Nonfiction Award, and The Third Coast Fiction Award. Natalie received an MFA from Warren Wilson College. She teaches writing in Portland, Oregon, and she is currently working on a novel.

Publications by Two Sylvias Press:

The Daily Poet:
Day-By-Day Prompts For Your Writing Practice
by Kelli Russell Agodon and Martha Silano (Print and eBook)

The Daily Poet Companion Journal (Print)

Fire On Her Tongue:
An Anthology of Contemporary Women's Poetry
edited by Kelli Russell Agodon and Annette Spaulding-Convy
(Print and eBook)

The Poet Tarot and Guidebook:
A Deck Of Creative Exploration (Print)

Community Chest
by Natalie Serber (Print)

Phantom Son
by Sharon Estill Taylor (Print and eBook)

What The Truth Tastes Like
by Martha Silano (Print and eBook)

landscape/heartbreak
by Michelle Peñaloza (Print and eBook)

Earth, Winner of the 2014 Two Sylvias Press Chapbook Prize
by Cecilia Woloch (Print and eBook)

The Cardiologist's Daughter
by Natasha Kochicheril Moni (Print and eBook)

She Returns to the Floating World
by Jeannine Hall Gailey (Print and eBook)

Hourglass Museum
by Kelli Russell Agodon (eBook)

Cloud Pharmacy
by Susan Rich (eBook)

Dear Alzheimer's: A Caregiver's Diary & Poems
by Esther Altshul Helfgott (eBook)

Listening to Mozart: Poems of Alzheimer's
by Esther Altshul Helfgott (eBook)

Crab Creek Review 30ᵗʰ Anniversary Issue
featuring Northwest Poets
edited by Kelli Russell Agodon and Annette Spaulding-Convy
(Print and eBook)

Please visit Two Sylvias Press (www.twosylviaspress.com) for
information on purchasing our print books, eBooks, writing tools,
and for submission guidelines for our annual chapbook prize.
Two Sylvias Press also offers editing services and manuscript
consultations.

Created with the belief
that great writing is good for the world.

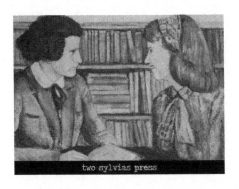

Visit us online: www.twosylviaspress.com

Also By NATALIE SERBER

Shout Her Lovely Name

Mothers and daughters ride the familial tide of joy, pride, regret, loathing, and love in these stories of resilient and flawed women. In a battle between a teenage daughter and her mother, wheat bread and plain yogurt become weapons. An aimless college student, married to her much older professor, sneaks cigarettes while caring for their newborn son. On the eve of her husband's fiftieth birthday, a pilfered fifth of rum, an unexpected tattoo, and rogue teenagers leave a woman questioning her place. And in a suite of stories, we follow capricious, ambitious single mother Ruby and her cautious, steadfast daughter Nora through their tumultuous life—stray men, stray cats, and psychedelic drugs—in 1970s California. Gimlet-eyed and emotionally generous, achingly real and beautifully written, these unforgettable stories lay bare the connection and conflict in families. *Shout Her Lovely Name* heralds the arrival of a powerful new writer.
(Houghton Mifflin Harcourt, 2012)

Achingly true to life when it comes to the many ways mothers and daughters grow together and apart, over and over again.
—*O, the Oprah Magazine*

Shout Her Lovely Name was a *New York Times* 100 Notable Books of 2012.

Made in the USA
Charleston, SC
21 December 2015